I0116403

Disclaimer: Always consult your physician/healthcare provider before beginning a new exercise program or making significant changes to your current physical activity, especially if you have existing health conditions or concerns.

Introduction

This booklet reminds the reader that

the **Heart**

is one of the most important organs in the body, pumping blood to **30 trillion cells** to keep them alive by providing essential food and oxygen. This booklet then describes a simple, easy-to-use, aerobic exercise program that will build the **strength and function** of your

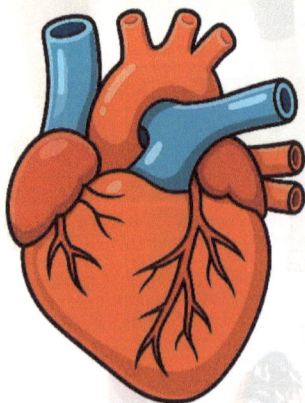

Exercising your
Heart <u>will</u>...

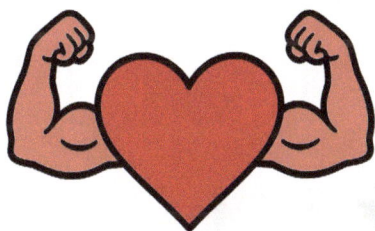

Strengthen your
Heart muscle[1]

Improve your
coronary circulation[2]

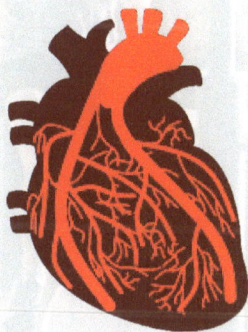

Activate/strengthen other **major organ systems** in your body[3,4]

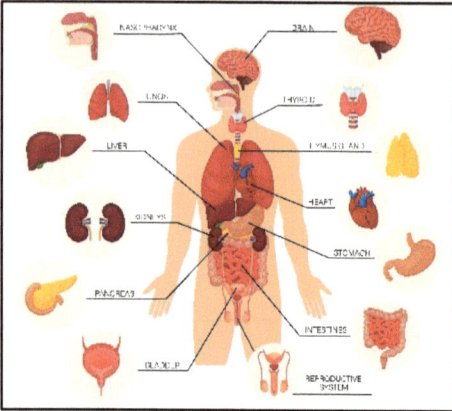

Improve your **cognitive (brain) function**[5,6]

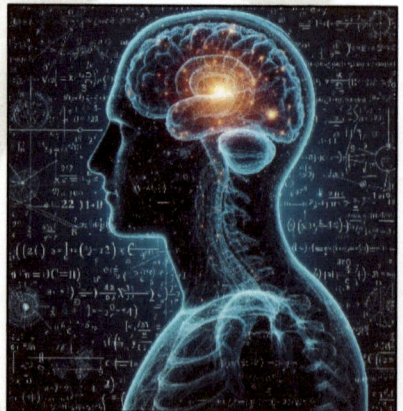

Increase your **lifespan**[7]

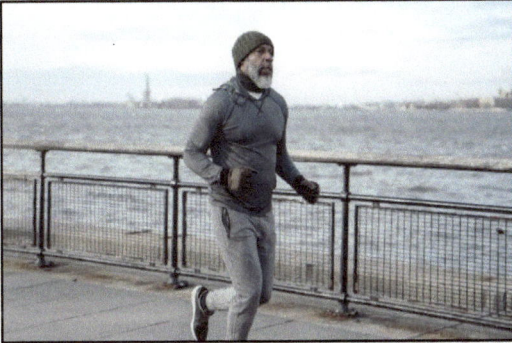

Reduce your acquiring many **common diseases** (diabetes, cancer, coronary, etc.)[8]

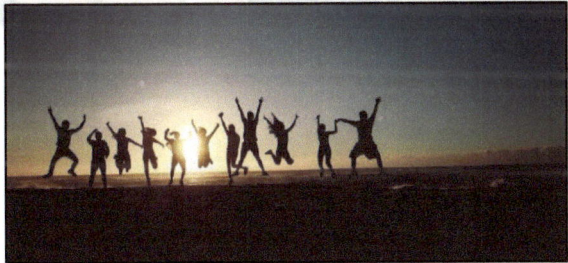

And these benefits will increase

your quality of life!

So, how do you exercise your

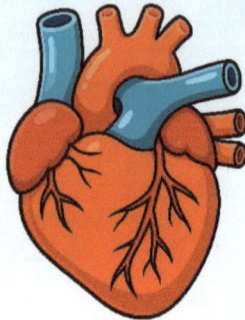

It's very easy …

1. Get your **Heart** **rate up!**

2. **Keep it up for** <u>**20– 30 minutes!**</u>

3. **Do this multiple times per week!**

Remember, your

Heart is a **muscle**, and exercise builds **strength and function** like it does with most other muscles in your body.

As you know, your arm muscles could go from this...

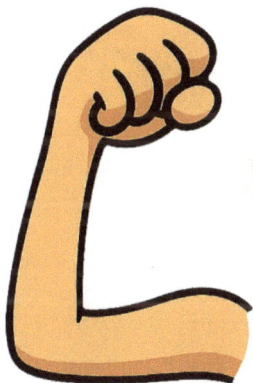

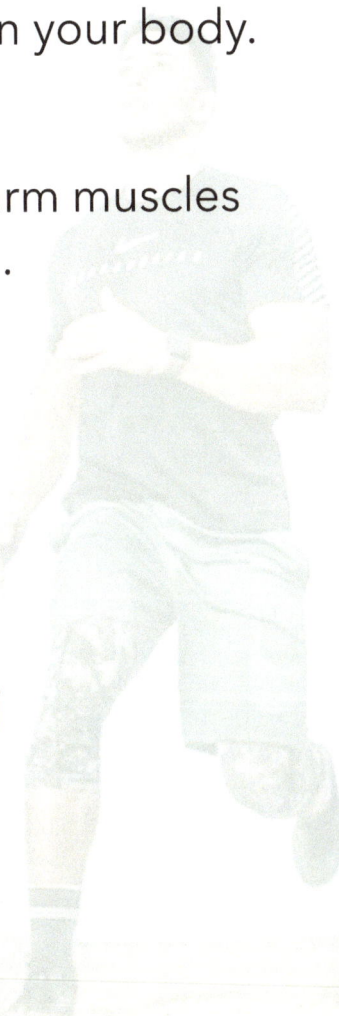

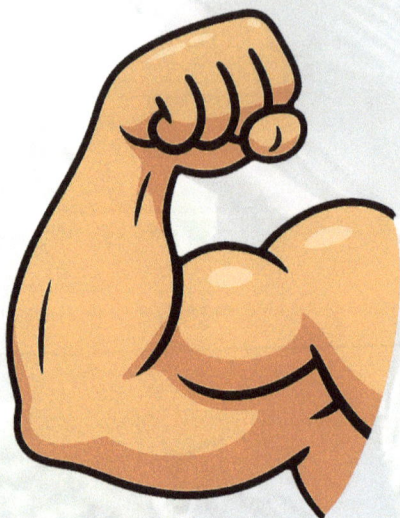

...to *this* with **exercise**

Uhhh... maybe not quite this much 🙁

The same applies

to your **Heart**

Aerobic exercise will increase its
Strength and Function!

Aerobic exercise is a physical activity
that …

uses large muscle groups, is
rhythmic and repetitive, and
increases your heart rate
and oxygen use.

Familiar examples of **aerobic exercise** are…

Boxing

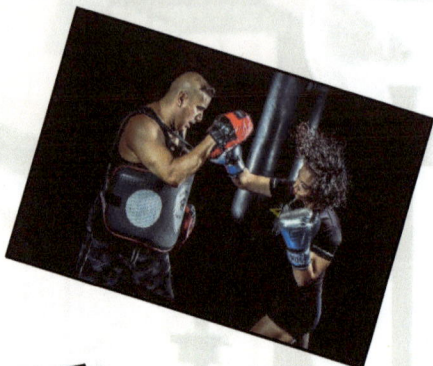

Swimming

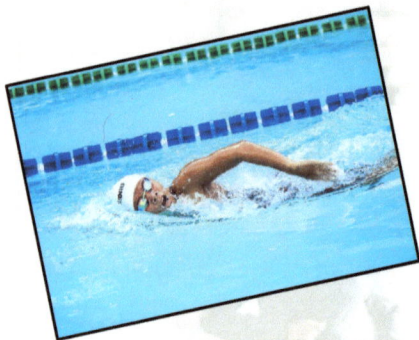

Hockey

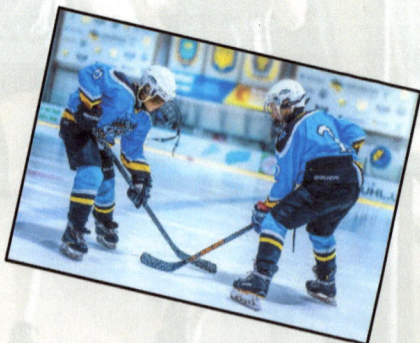

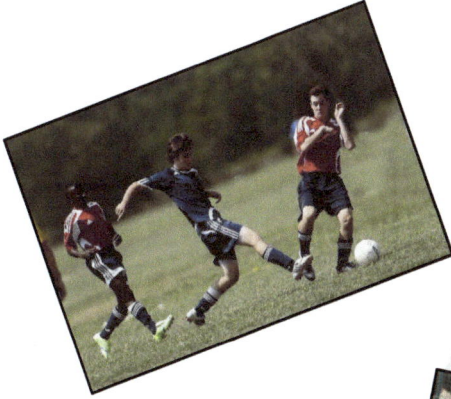

Soccer

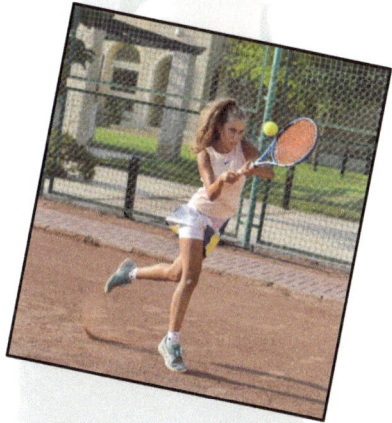

Tennis

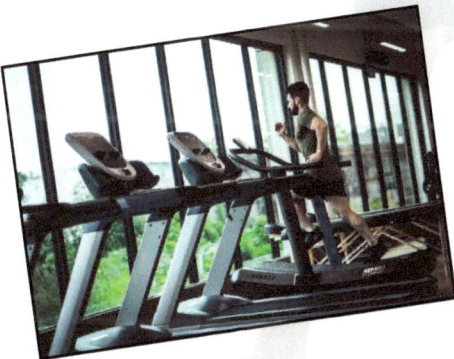

Treadmill

But these aerobic
exercises may
require expensive...

facilities,
equipment,
excessive time,
a team...

You **don't** have to use these
to **exercise your heart!**

You can exercise your **Heart** by

- ## RUNNING

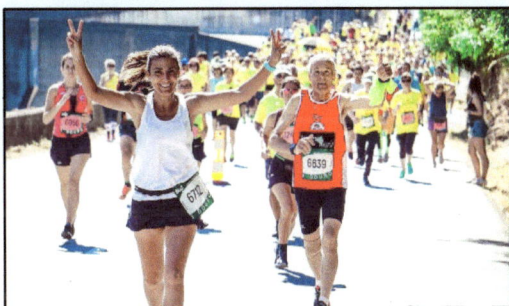

- ## JOGGING

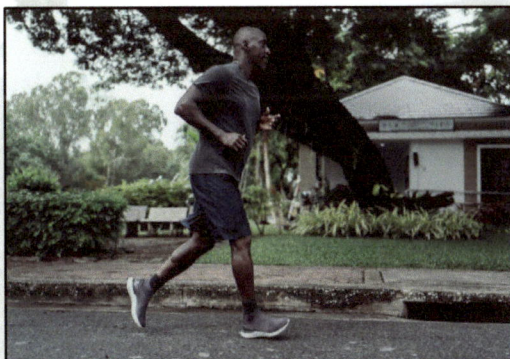

- **<u>WALKING</u>**[9]

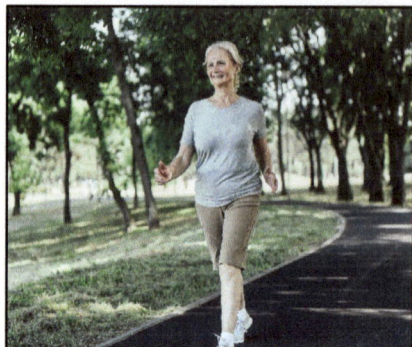

And, performed *correctly*, these aerobic exercises will…

get your
Heart
rate up!

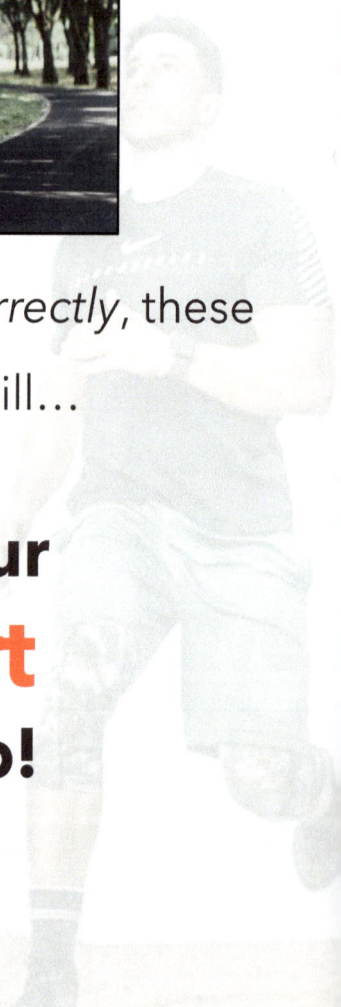

To **get started:**

Step 1: Check with your health care provider to see if you are physically ready to *safely begin* an **aerobic exercise** program. If your provider approves, then…

Step 2: Purchase a **Heart** rate watch:

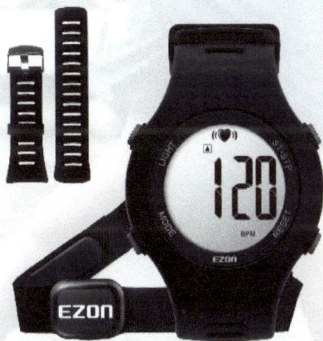

Purchase a watch that provides <u>continuous heart rate</u> measurements. For example, an EZON Heart Rate Monitor Watch and Strap can be purchased for about $40.

Step 3: Go for a walk, jog, or run (choose based on age and current physical condition).

IMPORTANTLY, move fast enough to get your **Heart** rate up *but* slow enough to keep moving for the **entire 20-30 minutes**.

Note (This is key): You must keep your heart rate up for *at least* 20-30 minutes each exercise session. Do this by controlling your pace (speed). As your heart rate goes up, slow down so you can keep moving for at least 20 minutes. Monitor your heart rate each exercise session to identify your approximate average rate for use in future sessions.

Step 4: Continue this exercise every 2 or 3 days for several weeks and keep track of your _average_ **Heart** rate for each exercise session.

When you are comfortable with your current exercise **Heart** rate, begin _moving a bit faster_ and note **_your_** new pace and average exercise **Heart** rate.

Your eventual **GOAL**?

An **increase** in average exercise **Heart** rate during your 20-30 minute aerobic exercise sessions.

For reference, the **predicted maximum exercise Heart** rate decreases with age[10] and yours can be calculated by subtracting **your age** from the number **220**.

For example…

- For a <u>20-year-old</u> the *average* maximum **Heart** rate is **~200 bpm.**

- For a <u>50-year-old</u> the *average* maximum **Heart** rate is **~170 bpm**.

- For an <u>80-year-old</u> the *average* maximum **Heart** rate is **~140 bpm.**

Note: These **maximum Heart** rates are based on population averages, and individual maximum **Heart** rates may be below or above these average values.

By comparing your **current**

exercise Heart rate to the

predicted maximum Heart

rate for your age, you will know

where you stand with your

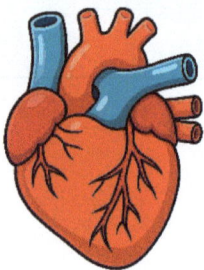

Strength and Function

And you will have strengthened your
lower body muscles as well!

It may take *many months* to reach your chosen goal, so **be patient!**

You will sleep and feel better knowing you have invested in getting and maintaining a **strong...**

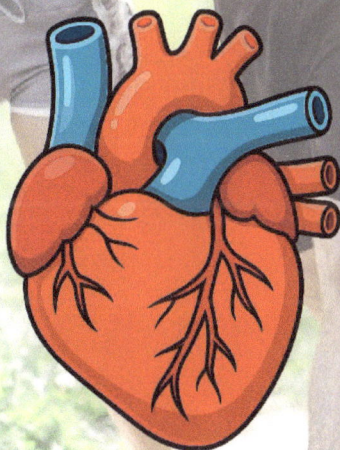

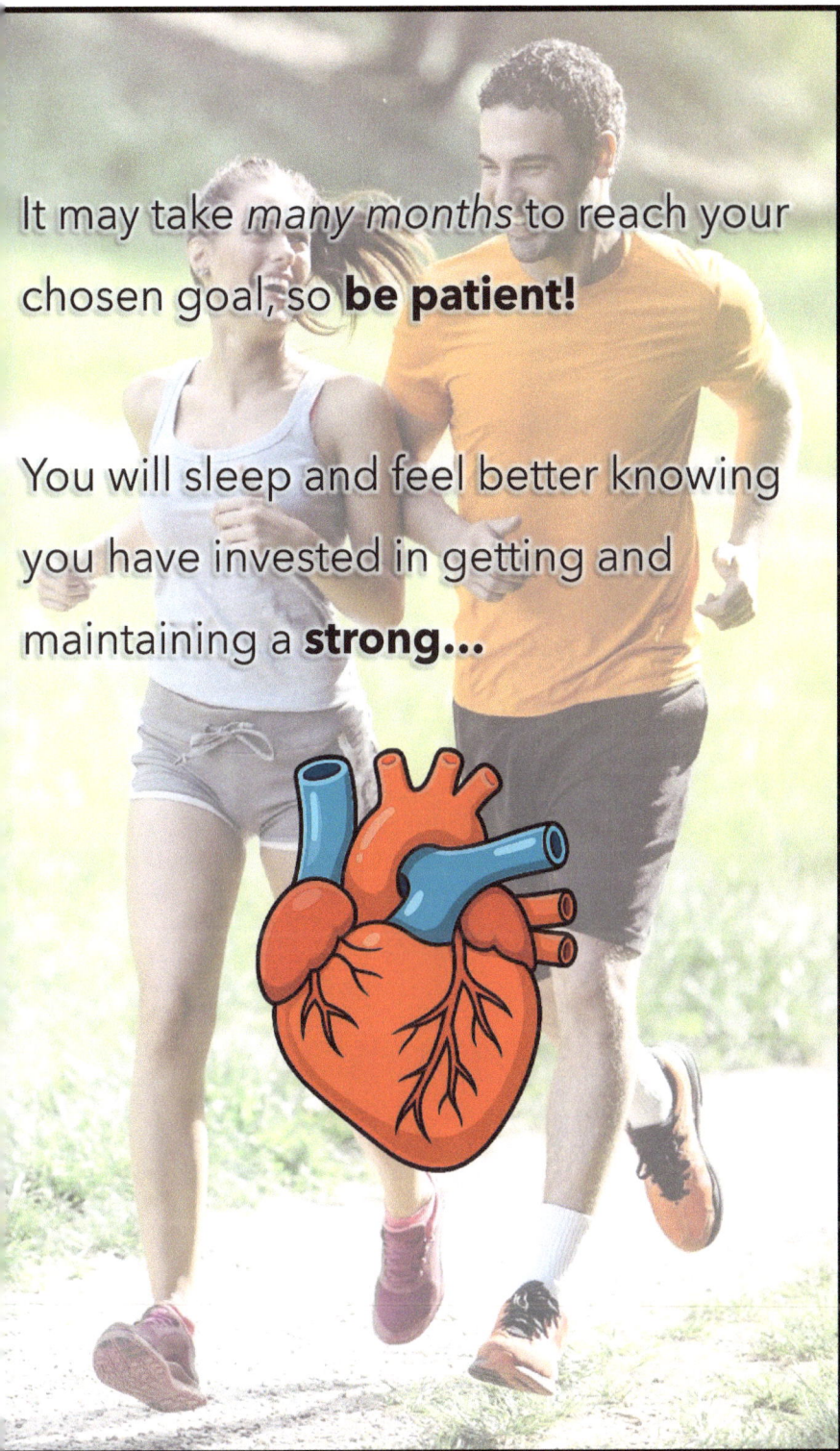

Bibliography

Note: Only a few of the thousands of relevant publications have been listed. The reader is encouraged to visit the National Library of Medicine online for additional references.

1. Short-term exercise-induced protection of cardiovascular function and health: why and how fast does the heart benefit from exercise? Dick H J Thijssen, Laween Uthman, Yasina Somani, Niels van Royen, J Physiol. 2022 Mar;600(6):1339-1355.

2. Exercise Training as a Mediator for Enhancing Coronary Collateral Circulation: A Review of the Evidence   Thomas Nickolay [1], Simon Nichols [2], Lee Ingle [3], Angela Hoye   Curr Cardiol Rev. 2020;16(3):212-220.

3. Association of Cardiorespiratory Fitness with Long Term Mortality among Adults Undergoing Exercise Treadmill Testing. K. Mandsager, S. Harb, P Cremer, D. Phelan, S. Nissen, W. Jaber JAMA Network Open 2018;1(6); e183605

4. Exercise, ageing and the lung M A Roman, H B Rossiter, R Casaburi European Respiratory J   2016 Nov;48(5):1471-1486.

5. Effects of Physical Exercise on Cognitive Functioning and Wellbeing: Biological and Psychological Benefits L Mandolesi, A Polverino, S Montuori, F Foti, G Ferraioli, P Sorrentino, G Sorrentino Front Psychol. 2018 Apr 27;9:509.

6. Effectiveness of exercise for improving cognition, memory and executive function: a systematic umbrella review and meta-meta-analysis Ben Singh, Hunter Bennett, Aaron Miatke, Dorothea Dumuid, Rachel Curtis, et al. bjsports-2024-10.1136, 108589

7. Lack of exercise is a major cause of chronic diseases. Booth FW, Roberts CK, Laye MJ. Compr Physiol 2012; 2:1143–1211.

8. Move more, age well: prescribing physical activity for older adults. J Thornton, W Morley, S Sinha. CAMJ January 27, 2025, 197 (3) E59-E67;

9. Daily walking and Mortality in Racially and Socioeconomically Diverse U.S. Adults Liu L,Guochong J, Shrubsole M, Wen W, Anderson S,Sudengo S, Zheng W. Am J Preventive Medicine 69; 4, October 2025

10. The Response of Healthy Men to Treadmill Exercise. Wolthuis, R.A., Froelicher, V.F., Fischer, J., and Triebwasser, J.H. Circulation, 55:153-157, 1977

The author is a Cardiovascular Scientist with degrees from Michigan and Michigan State Universities. He set up & managed the NASA Cardiovascular Laboratory supporting Apollo and Spacelab spaceflight programs, conducted extensive cardiovascular research on USAF aircrew at the School of Aerospace Medicine, served as Senior Scientist at Medtronic and Director of Product Development at Squibb Medical Systems. He subsequently led the startup & development of three medical device companies. He is a Fellow of the American College of Cardiology, the American Physiological Society and the Aerospace Medical Association. He lives in Woodinville, WA.

www.ingramcontent.com/pod-product-compliance
Lightning Source LLC
Chambersburg PA
CBHW041224270326

41933CB00001B/43

* 9 7 9 8 2 1 8 8 3 5 2 9 3 *